SURVIVAL SECRETS FOR THE NEW GRADUATE NURSE

ELENA MAZZELLA, RN, BSN

ISBN-13: 978-0692513880
ISBN-10: 0692513884

4

The alarm clock screams me awake at 5:00 in the morning. I leap out of bed, feeling short of breath. Did I wake up early enough? I don't want to be late. Today is my first day as a *registered nurse*. I have worked so hard to get here. I don't want to mess it up.

I get ready for work. I make sure my hair is pinned up, and my white scrubs are perfectly ironed. Patting myself down: black pens, check. Stethoscope, check. Pen light, check. Scissors, check. Notebook, check. I.D. badge, check. Keys, check. Wallet, check. Cell phone, check. Packed lunch, check. Water bottle, check. I walk out the front door and stand there for an extra minute, making sure I didn't forget anything.

I step into my car and drive to work. Where do I park? I hope my car is in the right parking area. I walk up the stairs to my unit paying careful attention to the signs and arrows on the walls. Wow, this place is a maze. I am here thirty minutes early. What do I do? Do I sit down? Do I just stand around the nurses' station? I sit down. Everyone is so busy running around, writing things down, looking at charts, darting in and out of patient rooms.

It is time to clock in. I follow the instructions on the paper I got during new employee orientation. Deep breath. Calm down, Elena. The charge nurse says hello, and lets me know my preceptor is running a few minutes late. I am sweating as I wait. I have no idea how this day is going to go or what my preceptor will expect of me.

"Hi, Elena!" I hear from across the nurses' station. I practically jump out of the chair... "Hi... good morning," I stutter. "I am glad that we met before the rush of today." She says sweetly with a compassionate smile, "Today you will just be observing me. Let's get started." I exhale a breath that I might have been holding for nearly ten minutes.

Observe. I can do that. Yes, let's get started on the first day of the rest of my nursing career.

My highest hope for this book is that reading it will help new graduate nurses become more prepared for success. Maybe they'll even use it in the future when they are ready to train a new graduate nurse themselves.

So here it goes (in no particular order or format).

Introduction

When I graduated nursing school, I still felt ill prepared to work as a nurse. Most new nurses feel the same way. There is a good reason for that feeling. The truth is, no new graduate nurse is ready to be on his or her own right away. This is why hospitals and other health care facilities generally have an orientation or preceptorship program for the new grad nurses they hire.

This short period of time in a nurse's career can be extremely formative. Nursing scholars have studied it extensively. There are many peer-reviewed journal articles in nursing literature that discuss the preceptorship process, the roles and relationships between experienced nurses and novice nurses, and what constitutes a successful program. Every new nurse will go through this initial training and orientation to the field; and even when it is over, they will still have much to learn. In truth, all nurses (even the most experienced nurses) are still learning. That is one of the best aspects of our line of work. We never stop learning.

I vividly remember my own preceptorship program, and I have successfully precepted a few new graduate nurses as well. I enjoy teaching and doing my part to welcome new nurses into this amazing field. However, there are twenty-four "survival secrets" I wish all new graduate nurses knew before starting. More importantly, I believe all new nurses would benefit from knowing them before entering such a program. Having this knowledge will save both parties involved a lot of valuable time and energy (trust me, a nurse really needs to conserve time and energy); prevent undue stress and anxiety (didn't you get enough of these in nursing school?); and possibly even prevent unnecessary tears (emotionally touching moments in nursing will bring enough of those in the future).

I am not an expert preceptor. I am not an experienced writer. This book will be littered with bias and my own opinions, and it will not reference nursing literature in APA format. It will not be peer reviewed or scientific in any way, but I am hoping that my peers will read it and enjoy it. I looked all over the internet for something that offered tips or advice for new graduate nurses in a preceptorship program, and I could not find anything other than disorganized dialogues in nursing forums. There seems to be a lot of information available for preceptors, and hardly anything at all for preceptees. So, I decided to write this very informal book.

SURVIVAL SECRET #1

Meet your preceptor before you start your preceptorship.

It is okay if you don't, but generally it is a good idea to meet your preceptor in person before you start your first day of training. Find out when they are on the schedule and go in to say hello. A simple introduction is really enough, but if they have a moment you can ask them a few questions you might need answered before starting.

SURVIVAL SECRET #2

Know your preceptor's schedule and exchange phone numbers.

Obviously, you will be required to work whatever days (or nights if you are working nights) your preceptor is working. Make sure you get a copy of their schedule from the very beginning. You don't want to be calling the charge nurses or director to find out when you are supposed to work. If there is a scheduling conflict that you cannot work around, let them know right away. Make sure you exchange phone numbers with them. A quick text to let them know you are running late, or to confirm a schedule date, or to clear something up that has been worrying you is always appreciated. Also, your preceptor may need to call out sick at some point and would need to let you know. You may need to be assigned to another nurse that day. It is simply a good idea to have a method of communication outside of work just in case.

SURVIVAL SECRET#3

Be on time.

Many nurses actually come in early to find out their patient assignment, look up labs and medications, and review doctor's orders before they even get a report from the off-going nurse. Other nurses (including myself) cut it close and punch in just in time to be considered on time. Ask your preceptor what they prefer. Regardless, *always* be on time. It really slows down the day to go over everything that was already discussed during shift report, or to go through the patients' test results twice. Your preceptor (and your employer) will really appreciate you being punctual.

SURVIVAL SECRET #4

Be prepared.

Pens. Penlight. Stethoscope. Scissors. A notebook (any size that works for you). These are the essentials. You will absolutely need a notebook to write down what you are learning. The new information will be coming at you fast throughout each day, and you will need to refer back to it often. Eventually, you won't need the notebook anymore; but for now, you do. When you start the day (in the hospital setting) you will also need a role of tape, alcohol swabs, medicine cups, and flushes. Be sure to get those items into your pockets before you start making rounds and passing medications.

SURVIVAL SECRET #5

Understand that your preceptor is extremely busy.

Your preceptor has a full patient assignment. In fact, some charge nurses might even give them the most challenging patients because they know you are available to help them. This means that in addition to your preceptor's normally hectic day and typical heavy workload, they are doing their best to teach you everything you need to know to be on your own in just a few weeks. Some shifts are crazier than others. Be patient with them, help rather than hinder, and watch closely as your preceptor navigates the tornado shifts that you will certainly soon be gracefully handling on your own.

SURVIVAL SECRET #6

Ask a lot of questions. Especially the ones that make you feel stupid.

Preceptors worry if a preceptee does not ask questions. Asking questions is crucial in the learning process. It can be anything. "Is this the right form?" "Did I document this properly?" "Is this a stage I or a stage II pressure ulcer?" "Who is that doctor?" Ask the questions so that you know the answers because in nursing, not knowing the answer can be dangerous. You might feel stupid, and that is okay. I knew a nurse that did not know how to open the crash cart. She knew she was already supposed to know that, so she didn't ask because she felt embarrassed. Can you imagine how much more embarrassed she was during her first code blue? Exactly. Ask all of your questions, no matter what.

SURVIVAL SECRET #7

Write down key information and step-by-steps.

For example, if your preceptor teaches you how to use new equipment step-by-step, you'll want to write it down so that you can refer back to it when you're doing it without your preceptor over your shoulder. Write down the codes for any locked rooms you need to enter throughout the day rather than asking for the same code over and over. Writing new information down will help you to remember it and save you time. As I mentioned before, eventually you will not need this notebook at all and everything will become second nature to you, but that takes time.

SURVIVAL SECRET #8

Tell your preceptor what your weak points were in nursing school.

This gives them a good idea of what skills they need to help you strengthen. It is your responsibility to make sure you are filling in the knowledge gaps and honing your skills. It is essential for you to know your own weaknesses and communicate your goals throughout the preceptorship. Your weak points can be very broad (e.g. general assessment skills, medications) or very specific (e.g. how to start an IV, how to read doctor's orders).

SURVIVAL SECRET #9

Some of what you learned in school is different from the "real world"
of nursing.

Try to keep an open mind. I won't go into great detail on this one. You will see. If there is a faster, more efficient way to do something, a nurse will find it.

SURVIVAL SECRET #10

Trust yourself.

You did graduate nursing school and then passed the NCLEX, right? Although there is still a lot to learn, you should be confident in what you know. It is okay to ask for confirmation for a while, but eventually you just need to trust your knowledge. This self-trust is important. You will need it when you have to stand your ground and advocate for your patients.

SURVIVAL SECRET #11

You aren't expected to know all of the meds.

Despite what your pharmacology professor led you to believe, *no nurse* knows the generic and trade names, indications, side effects, drug-drug interactions and adverse effects of every medication. That is why we have drug guides. Eventually, you will become familiar with the drugs you see every day. However, you are absolutely expected to know every medication before you administer it. Bring a drug guide, download a drug guide app to your phone, or know how to use your facility's drug guide… then look it up like the rest of us do.

SURVIVAL SECRET #12

Do not pretend to know something if you don't know it.

Part One

And never say that you have done something if you haven't. Preceptors know that you will not always get every skill perfected in nursing school clinicals because the opportunities often just don't arise. If you have never inserted a urinary catheter for a female or male patient; if you have never started an IV; if you have never given an IM injection; if you have never completed real life tracheostomy care (or any other skill) just say so when you are asked. Even better, tell your preceptor right away that you need those experiences. You are not going to be penalized for not knowing. Nursing students are becoming increasingly limited in what they are allowed to do during clinical rotations often because of the college or the hospital policies.

Part Two

If a patient or family member asks you something that you do not know, say, "I don't know, but I can find out for you" or something of the like. Do not ever guess or make something up. This can be very confusing for patients, and it will make you look bad when they find out the real answers. You will come off as far more intelligent when you demonstrate how quickly you can find the answers for them and provide them with accurate information. This still happens to me on the daily basis at work. These are learning moments not only for your patient but for you as well. And, in the future, when you get asked the same question, you will know the answer!

SURVIVAL SECRET #13

Develop an organizational system/checklist that works for you.

Every nurse carries notes and a checklist around with them all day. They create it in the morning and then add to it and check off items throughout the shift. There is an example of a template that I have used since I started working as a nurse at the end of this book. At work, I hand draw the boxes on a blank sheet of paper every morning and everything is hand written. However, for the sake of legibility I created a table and typed out some things that I might write. By the end of a shift this paper looks like a jumbled mess of disorganized scribble from all the little notes I jot down, circle, cross out and check off; but it works (for me).

Every nurse I have trained adopted this method, but that does not mean it is the best method. What is important is that it works for you, and it keeps you organized and on task. Some other nurses that I have worked with keep a separate sheet of paper for each patient, or they carry a binder or a clipboard. Your preceptor is likely using a system that has worked for them for years. Try it and see if you like it. Check out what the other nurses are using. You can also create your own, or tweak someone else's to suit your needs. Being organized is integral to staying on task and managing time efficiently.

SURVIVAL SECRET #14

Introduce yourself to the patients.

It is okay to be shy or timid at first, but at the very least you should say hello with a smile and tell patients your name. "Hi (patient name here) my name is (your name here), it's nice to meet you. I am a nurse, and I'll be working with (preceptor name here) today." I like to jokingly tell patients that they are getting the two for one nurse special. It always lightens the mood and alleviates their apprehension to be taken care of by a new nurse. I mean, put yourself in their shoes. You just had surgery, you are in a lot of pain, and you need dressing changes and lots of IV medications. How would you feel if you had a newbie nurse? Be empathetic and kind. Showing them how much you care goes a long, long way.

SURVIVAL SECRET #15

Pay close attention during shift report.

This is one of the most vital few minutes of a nurse's day. The information handed off in report enables continuity of patient care. Your preceptor expects you to know this and pay attention. At first, a lot of the words, abbreviations, procedures, acronyms, etc. might worry you. You will be thinking, "Am I supposed to know this? I should have brought my textbook. I have no idea what that nurse just said." Don't let your worry of not knowing what is being said distract you from listening. This new language of nursing will soon become easier to speak than your native language. Just remember: ask questions!

SURVIVAL SECRET #16

You are not expected to have perfected time management.

Even when nurses are done with orientation, they usually still need to work on time management a little bit. You might be wondering if you will ever clock out at a reasonable time. Don't worry. You will get there. Make small time goals for yourself while you are training. For instance, "I will be done passing morning medications by 10 am."

SURVIVAL SECRET #17

Take your break and eat lunch (and stay hydrated).

What would you do if your patient did not eat or drink anything and did not produce any urine for twelve hours? You would likely be administering an IV fluid bolus, checking their vitals, having blood labs drawn, and assessing for reasons for the decrease in appetite and fluid intake. I don't need to tell you that being dehydrated and not urinating are bad for your health, your performance, your brain power, your kidneys (and so on). You are a nurse. You know this. Bring a water bottle, buy a water bottle, drink from the water fountain. Drink, drink, drink!

There will *always* be something that you need to do. If all of your patients are stable, stop yourself. I mean really force yourself to stop what you are doing and sit down to take your break. There is an obscene amount of research on the negative health effects of not taking a break at work, and obviously not eating or drinking anything for twelve plus hours is not good for you. I know a lot of nurses who do not eat lunch or take a break. Your preceptor might be one of them. DO NOT adopt that habit. Take care of yourself.

SURVIVAL SECRET # 18

Ask other nurses if they have anything for you to learn/practice.

It is impossible to practice all of the skills you will learn as a nurse in just a few weeks. To maximize your opportunities, ask the other staff if they have something you can do. In one shift, your preceptor might not have anything that is new for you, but your coworkers might have a cardiac IV drip, blood transfusions, new IV starts, central line removal or dressing change, and so on. Take advantage of those learning opportunities. The nurse that lets you do it for them will appreciate the help as well.

SURVIVAL SECRET #19

Be helpful and kind to the PCAs / CNAs.

You will *not* survive if the PCAs / CNAs do not respect you. You can gain their respect in four major ways: 1. Express how extremely appreciative you are of their hard work, and how much they help you throughout the shift. Do this every single shift. 2. Don't delegate a task to them that you have time to do yourself. They are busy too. 3. Do what they do. Jump in to help them clean that patient that was incontinent bowel and is so covered in it that the situation seems impossible. 4. When you do need to delegate to them, say please, ask them nicely if they are able to get to it, and say thank you. If they aren't able to get to it, either try to manage it yourself or ask another PCA. If you have a good relationship with your assistants, they will not mind doing something for a patient that is not part of their assignment. Trust me, a good relationship with your assistants will save you on the regular basis. A bad one will make your job miserable.

SURVIVAL SECRETS #20

Overcome your fear of physicians.

Some physicians are incredibly humble and actually love to teach nurses or anyone who will listen. Some are more approachable than others. Some are downright mean and disrespectful. Regardless, do not be intimidated by them. Yes, they went to medical school, and they have more medical knowledge than you do. They make a lot more money than you. And, of course, they give you orders. No matter what, they are still just people with regular lives (albeit sometimes fancier ones), families, and problems. Introduce yourself to them so they know your face and name. Let them know you are new to the staff. You will be calling them more than you can imagine. Eventually, there will be a level of trust and even friendship between you and the physicians you work with regularly. When you do come across a rude physician, just let it roll off your shoulders and notify your supervisor of their behavior. Honestly, physicians treating nurses poorly is rare nowadays. I can't remember the last time a physician was disrespectful to me. Of course, a lot of this depends on the culture that is established by the facility.

SURVIVAL SECRET #21

Communicate with your preceptor if you are completely overwhelmed.

If you feel like your head is spinning, you are about to cry, or you are about to have a full-blown panic attack, please tell your preceptor! They will work with you to make modifications to the training that will hopefully prevent you from feeling that way. Also, sometimes you might just have to trust them. I have had a preceptee come to me and say, "I feel like I am drowning right now." I went over what they had already done so far, what they had not done, and how much time they had left in the shift. Then, my response was "You are not drowning, you are fine. Just keep going." Part of feeling as though you are never going to get everything done is the fact that you do not have time management down pat yet. You aren't yet able to accurately assess how much time it is going to take you to get a certain thing done, get in and out of each patient room, finish your charting, etc. Again, I promise, you will get there.

SURVIVAL SECRET #22

Understand your preceptor's role in the relationship.

There is a ton of nursing literature available about the role of a nurse preceptor. Read a few articles so that you have a general idea of what your preceptor should be doing as well as what they are experiencing. If an experienced nurse who has never been a preceptor before is training you, try to be patient with them. That might be you one day.

SURVIVAL SECRET #23

It is okay to fire your preceptor.

After a week or two into the preceptorship, you might feel like your preceptor is just not a good match. If this occurs, first try to talk to your preceptor about it. Sometimes it can be related to a simple misunderstanding or miscommunication. In general, the need to "fire" a preceptor can happen for a lot of reasons. Sometimes there is just a personality clash; sometimes their teaching methods do not work for the preceptee and they are not good at adapting their methods for different types of learners; and sometimes a preceptor just might not be cut out for the role. You have every right to switch to a different preceptor if necessary. If talking to your preceptor doesn't work, let your supervisor know.

SURVIVAL SECRET #24

Be the real you.

You may feel a bit like an outsider at first. That is because working long shifts together and going through seemingly impossible situations as a team creates a bond much like a family. You are a new member of that family, and they need to get to know you. You will laugh with them and cry with them. You will help each other through challenges both professional and personal. You will be celebrating many holidays, birthdays, baby showers, sendoffs, weddings, and accomplishments with them. Let them get to know you. Build trust and friendship. Let your patients get to know you, too. No nurse wants to work with a robot, and no patient wants to be cared for by one, either. Remember, caring for others is always personal.

I drive to work, park, walk into my unit and clock in as if on autopilot. I don't get lost in the hospital maze anymore. It is an ideal morning; all of the patients are stable. I join into the nursing station chatter about nothing in particular; laughing and hugging the nurses I haven't seen in a while. My work family. The night nurses give me report on my six patients, and we exchange words about the patients' care plans, if plans are appropriate, and what needs to be done for them today. I am speaking a nursing language I never thought I would learn. I sit down to review charts, orders, meds, and patient data.

A new graduate nurse comes up to me as I stand up and nervously says, "Hi, my name is Kerry, you are going to be my preceptor starting next week." This is surreal. It wasn't long ago that I said those exact words. I smile. "It's so great to meet you, Kerry. I look forward to working with you next week. I have never been a preceptor before, so we are in this together. I'm sure we will do great." I'm not sure. I've read a bunch of articles about being a preceptor, but like anything else, there is a huge difference between reading about it and doing it. I do remember my own preceptorship and how I felt as a new graduate nurse. I do know now what I wish I knew then. So, I'll start with that. It is the beginning of a new chapter in my nursing career, and I am privileged to be a part of Kerry's first page.

Pt Room # / Last name	Pt Room # / Last name
Vitals 0800: ACHS 1200: Bgl:__ 1600: Bgl:__ Abnormal labs: BNP 898, Na 128 WBC 22 To do list: ☐IV antibiotic administration ☑CXR (☐follow up on results) ☑Heart failure education	Vitals 0800: 1200: 1600: Abnormal labs: Hemoglobin 7.9 To do list: ☑ Stool collection for occult ☑ CT Abdomen/Pelvis ☐PRBC transfusion (2 units) ☐EGD/Colonoscopy procedure
Pt Room # / Last name	Pt Room # / Last name
Vitals Q4Neuro✓s 0800: ☑0800 1200: ☐1200 1600: ☐1600 Abnormal labs: INR 1.8 To do list: ☐PTT level 1600 (heparin gtt) ☑MRI Brain ☐Coumadin diet education ☑Stroke education	Vitals ACHS 0800: Bgl:__ 1200: Bgl:__ 1600: Abnormal labs: none To do list: ☐OOB to chair post op ☑follow up with case manager ☐Physical Therapy consult ☑Med education: morphine ☐Advance clears to full liquid
Pt Room # / Last name	Pt Room # / Last name
Vitals 0800: 1200: 1600: Abormal labs: K 3.3, BUN 38, Creatinine 2.6 To do list: ☐Strict I &Os ☐Replace potassium ☑ Collect wound culture ☐Central line dressing change ☑Contact isolation education ☑Wound care nurse consult	Vitals 0800: 1200: 1600: Abnormal labs: WBC 24, Mg 1.6 To do list: ☑Collect urine specimen ☐Replace magnesium ☑discontinue urinary catheter ☑void post catheter removal

www.ingramcontent.com/pod-product-compliance
Lightning Source LLC
Chambersburg PA
CBHW060516210326
41520CB00015B/4231